ANGELOLOGY

A Better Connection with Universal Mind

Invite your Angels, Ancestors and Tribe to heal with you.

With Helpful Natural ways to Increase Immunity and Health

Published by:

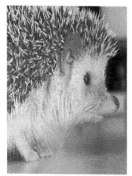

Healing Hedgehog Press
Cupertino, California   95014

healingangelguides@yahoo.com
Email us today.

Web Site with TV shows, trainings, and testimonials.
www.healingangelguides.com
(408) 253-6577 Office Phone

Copyright ©2008 through 2014, by Paul Barbaro, Your Health is Your Wealth Foundation, and Saint Joseph Healing Foundation, St. Jude's Healing Foundation, Embassy of the Kingdom of God, and Heart to Heart Healing Center, Cupertino, California 95014.

You may copy and pass out this book based on certain conditions. Please see the permission available to copy this book in the back of this book. This is extremely generous of the author to grant this permission to copy.

Our Heart Ribbon Logo on the back cover is our branding communication identity to the world. This logo is copyrighted in all it's forms, alterations, manipulations, color combinations, re-sizing, animating, "3-D–ing," including any digital or manual shape changing, background colors, textures, stripes, shapes, step and repeat, additions or deletions of number of ribbons or hearts, etc., and all other combinations of artistic variations, alterations and changes. This is because we have tried hundreds of color combinations shapes, ribbon widths, heart shapes, colors, styles, textures, etc. and all of these trials and errors are our intellectual properties. If one must altar, please submit the alterations to us for approval or rejection. This will save one a lot of work and headaches.

All United States and international rights reserved.

UCC 1-308, et al.

First Edition

ISBN-13: 978-1496132178

ISBN-10: 1496132173

BISAC: Health & Fitness / Healing

You Can Learn to Communicate with Your Angels and Spiritual Realm

The suggestions in this book do help one to make a better connection to and with their spiritual realm. One simply reads the suggestions and does them and then remain quiet enough to "see" "feel" the results. This is not an instant action. It may require many asks. Be persistant and insistant and connection will be made.

Editors Note: One can see FREE training videos of this technique at www.healingangelguides.com/ Please click on "Training" and watch these videos with a friend or partner, read this book together and then take turns doing this process on each other, One can get a result while doing the exercises. The gains can be tremendous.

Youtube Videos that You can watch Online:

Youtube address for Video #1:
http://www.youtube.com/watch?v=M_CdVe-_qsY

Youtube address for Video #2:
http://www.youtube.com/watch?v=FE-aNtbuqlk

Youtube address for Video #3:
http://www.youtube.com/watch?v=XunCrduVOto

Other Books by Paul Barbaro

Heart to Heart Healing – Getting Rid of Early Childhood Trauma. When you care enough to make a difference in a loved one's health. This early trauma creates an energy imbalance which can cause illness. This technique resolves that conflicted energy over time. It is just like a battery running out of energy through attached jumper cables.

Healing Our Community – Real Healing for our communities and for our nation.

Tribal Healing Sets You Free – Heal Your Tribe, Heal Your Energy, Heal Your Life.

Healing Our Company – Team Building that Heals. Real Healing for a Troubled Workplace.

Two Shamans and a Healer – The Quest for a Healing Discovery and, An Outline for a PBS Special

The Lightbearer's Handbook – Let Your Healing Light Shine Brighter

Disclaimer

Required Disclaimer: The information provided in this book is for educational and entertainment purposes only and is not intended to diagnose, prevent, cure, nor treat any disease or condition. It is not intended as a substitute for competent medical care or advice. If one has pain or other health conditions then one is advised to see a medical professional immediately. If one is under a doctor's care, one must get their doctors permission to receive these energy healing processes. The information provided herein should not be construed as a health-care diagnosis, treatment regimen or any other prescribed health-care advice or instruction. The information is provided with the understanding that the publisher and author is not engaged in the practice of medicine or any other health-care profession and does not enter into a health-care practitioner/patient relationship with its readers. The publisher and author do/does not advise or recommend to its readers treatment or action with regard to matters relating to their health or well-being other than to suggest that readers consult appropriate health-care professionals in such matters. No action should be taken based solely on the content of this publication. The information and opinions provided herein are believed to be accurate and sound at the time of publication, based on the best judgment available to the author. However, readers who rely on information in this publication to replace the advice of health-care professionals, or who fail to consult with health-care professionals, assume all risks of such conduct. The publisher and author is/are not responsible for errors or omissions.

These statements have not been evaluated by the Food and Drug Administration. This product or process is not intended to diagnose, treat, cure, or prevent any disease.

If one has pain then one is advised to see a medical professional immediately. If one is under a doctor's care, one must get their doctor's permission to receive these energy healing processes. Pain is symptomatic. Always seek medical advice from your physician or other qualified healthcare provider for any questions one may have regarding any medical condition including pain. And under no circumstances discontinue taking any prescribed medications without your doctor's permission. There are life threatening major diseases and medical conditions that have no symptoms at all. Regularly scheduled medical checkups are extremely valuable.

More Disclaimer: I, Paul Barbaro, created this spiritual work is a complement to conventional medicine and alternative healing methods. I'm a minister and this spiritual energy work is not a substitute for conventional medical treatment of any kind, physical or psychological. For such issues you should seek the proper licensed physician or qualified health care professional. This energy work may help the bio-field to come into energetic balance. Qigong theory believes when one's energy field is in balance, the body's latent healing ability can heal itself. I make no promises nor guarantees about the results of this work. I am very grateful for this opportunity to work with everyone interested in healing. I, Paul Barbaro, make absolutely no promises, because every body is different and everybody responds differently to healing energy. "Viva la difference."

Revival of Ancient Traditional "Hands on Healing" Method

One thousand years ago when someone was sick they would go to the village square and the people of the village would form a circle around the sick person and place their hands on the person for half an hour or more. The person who was sick would get better. In this tradition healing is a tribal event.

Notice: This healing method revives the ancient and traditional "hands-on healing method" as spoken of in the Jewish sacred writings and in the Christian Bible, and uses the Buddhist, Hindu, Vedic, and Judeo-Christian teachings and upon the religious teachings of: "Do unto others as you would have them do unto you." It is also based on Chinese Ti-Chi, the movement of energy, and on Qui Gong, and other Asian and First American Nation (American Indian) energy religious and spiritual practices. Heart to Heart Healing University, Cupertino, California, is an ecclesiastic* educational association organized under the authority of the First Amendment of the Original Constitution for the United States, of the year of Our Lord 1789. This University is religious, it is a church university, and these healing processes are religious because they resolve spiritual stuck energy as well as the cellular memory of early physical trauma. All First Amendment rights are asserted, reserved, and protected herewith by this Notice, assertion, proclamation, and publication. The University is non-medical, non-denominational, and non-political. It is open to all races, creeds and religions, as well as to all sexual orientations.

This healing University is not exclusive nor discriminatory. This is because we all can use some healing.

Note: These processes are not instant. There are no magic bullets. There are no magic pills.

As Rome was not built in a day, and as your immune system is/was not instantly compromised, so these processes take time and work to achieve long lasting results. You and your partner are worth the work. You both are worth the time spent, and you are both worth working toward the results.

No claims of results can ever be made from these processes because every body and every trauma is different, and heals differently. Some chronic pain does not respond to balanced energy, one is always free to explore other avenues of healing.

Just for clarity, there is no suggestion that there is anything wrong with the reader, their families nor friends, nor any of our societies. We are all made perfectly. There is nothing wrong with you or anyone or anything else. To judge this would be an injustice to the judged. This authors goal is to help "Turn up the/your 'Light' a little brighter." Not that it's dim. Thank you for your understanding.

This healing method and these processes are not based on the belief systems of either the giver nor the receiver. This healing method operates at the cellular level. It can repair damaged nerve connections at the cellular level. It can repair/forgive past ancestor's health issues. Past DNA programming can be changed. This is good news for the pain sufferer. Recent scientific discoveries have proven that DNA and past trauma can be scessfully be reprogrammed. This healing can bring relief to the sufferer. There is hope.

Table of Contents

What's in it for me? Why should I care? .... Page 7

How to Ask Your Angels for what You Want ... Page 9

The Power of Honoring Your Ancestors .... Page 15

Angels in the Hospital .... Page 16

Angels in the Corporation .... Page 17

Angels in the Cubicle .... Page 19

Frequently Asked Questions (FAQ's) .... Page 21

Should Ask Questions (SAQ's) ,.................... Page 23

Prove to Me that Cell Memory is Real .... Page 25

The Love Never Dies .... Page 27

Bonus Book #2, Natural Health Tips .... Page 29

Section Two: A Bonus Separate Book

"What did they do 100 years ago before they had all these 'Miracle Drugs?'"

Helpful Natural Tips to Stay Healthy

Table of Contents for Bonus Book #2

Rescue & Strengthen Your Compromised
Immune System .... Page 31

A Gelatin Recipe to Handle Joint Pain .... Page 35

Improved Memory and Brain Performance ...... Page 37

A One Million Dollar Cash Savings .... Page 41

Bob Hope on Living to 100 Years Old .... Page 43

An Angel Story .... Page 45

Breakfast at McDonald's .... Page 47

A Story that Creates Hope .... Page 51

The Cost of a Miracle .... Page 57

How to Search Google for Health Information .. Page 61

Cancer and Major Diseases .... Page 63

More Cancer Notes .... Page 69

Dr. Emoto's Messages from Water .... Page 77

Labels for Water Bottles .... Page 80

How Can I Tell If I Am Dehydrated? .... Page 81

How the Buddha Achieved Enlightenment .... Page 83

Healing Principals .... Page 89

How to Re-Colonize Your Gut .... Page 92

Handling Your Enemies with Feng Shui .... Page 95

Working on a PBS Special .... Page 99

Bio of Author, Paul Barbaro .... Page 101

Angels 101, What You Need to Know:

Q: What's in it for me? And why should I care about Angels?

A: Please read this testimonial:
From: Linda H., Feb. 2012: "Everything in my life was falling apart, because everything I touched turned to crap. I was so tired of my life that I was suicidal. I met Paul at a New Year's Eve party, 2011, and he asked, "Of course you ask your angels for what you want... Don't you?" I could not believe my ears and I shouted: "Do you really believe that crap?" I emptied out the room we were in!

Paul calmly said: "I understand your feelings because there is so much misinformation about angels and spiritual things out there." "And he asked me to ask my angels to show me a sign that they are there."

"So I figured I had nothing to lose. For several nights after going to bed I asked my angels to show me that they are there, because I was certain that they weren't. Three days later in a dreamy state my angels came to me and told me that I was loved and cherished, and cared for, and that I was precious to them, and that they were always there for me, and if I needed anything I should just ask.

I was besides myself with amazement because I was a huge skeptic. Ever since then I have asked several times and my life has gone from crap to miracles.

To this day in November, 2012 the miracles continue."

"Thank you Paul for this information, my life is so much easier now. You are the Angel man."

- Linda H. from Walnut Creek, California.

Authors Note: I saw Linda H. in February 2014, and she is still in communication with her angels and with her spiritual realm and she says her life is fine. Enough said.

How to Ask your Angels for What You Want:

Each book in this healing series has information for making your life much easier by improving your energy and health, and that includes your spiritual life and health as well. This is a practical guide, one reads it and can immediately put this information to work in their life, and get a positive outcome! The results of 40 years of healing research is in this book, years of testing wrong answers, years of dialog with "experts" that had no clue. This book saves you years of re-inventing the wheel, and the cost of research. Here is the real and true information about Angels. Just try it for yourself. This author expects people to be skeptical at first. Everything here works very well:

Step # 1: Call your Angels, Guides, Masters, Ancestors, and friends/family to be present before you.* this author calls them "Your Gathering." Tell them you have requests for them and you need them to do these things for you immediately. Get their agreement to do this for you. They are there to help you and to protect you. So it is okay to ask them of these things. Then thank all of them for protecting you in the past, and for keeping you safe.

* There is no time nor space on the other side. All of life and all beings are present with you now. This is called simply: "Now."

This is a hard concept for we earthlings to grasp because we live so much in time and space. We created the concepts of time and space. Our rent and bills make this concept very real. My constant prayer is for me/us is to stop creating a time and space separation between myself/yourself and all other beings. This prayer includes God, Jesus, the Angels, Father Abraham, Moses, Buddha and all other beings. If I take a year to really master this concept and "I get it," That would be time well spent.

A Good Book says "Ask and you will receive." It doesn't say "Maybe," or "If you stand on your head for a month." Or "Do ___"X, do ___Y, and do ___Z," or anything else. If you just "get" and live just this one point, then you've got a thousand times the value of this book. Please write to this author if you have any issues with integrating this concept.

An important Key: Angels speak in pictures. If you are waiting for a descending cloud, a lightning bolt, a burning bush, a booming voice out of the clouds, you are sadly mistaken by Hollywood. Angels speak in pictures. You have to be quiet enough to hear or see these pictures. Very rarely will you hear a voice. Sometimes a total stranger will walk up to you and blurt out an answer that you have been needing for a long time, and then simply walk away, or disappear. That's a clue.

Step # 2: Tell your Gathering, verbatim: "My mind seems to be a movie projector running 24/7 out of control. Please stop all of this noise right now, and forever so I can think and focus clearly."

Step # 3: Tell your Gathering, verbatim: "I want you all to filter all information coming to me right now and forever, and I want you to only give me the information that is true and valid." "I haven't got time to re-invent the wheel, so you do this for me." Note: Please ask as many times as it takes to get the results you want.
Be sure to thank them in advance for doing this for you.

Step # 4: Then tell your Gathering, verbatim: "I want all of you to go through my subconscious mind and quiet all the disempowering thoughts that are holding me back from my full power to Be, Do and Have my full power as a spiritual being, and to do the work I was sent here to do." Be sure to thank them in advance for doing this for you. Say "Thank you all for all that you have done for me in the past and for covering my back, I really need you to do this for me now."

Step # 5: Then tell your Gathering, verbatim: "I want you-all to go through my body right now, and heal everything that needs to be healed. Including my brain! If you can't heal my body right now than tell me NOW, and clearly what I must do now to heal."

Note: This may include forgiveness of those that have wronged you. Brace yourself for that possibility. Be sure to thank them in advance for doing this for you.

Step # 6: Then tell your Gathering, verbatim: "For what purpose was I born?" and "Why am I here?" "I need the answer to this in the next forty-eight hours!" Be sure to thank them in advance for doing this for you.

Step # 7: Gratitude here is important. You say to them:

"Thank You Angels and Guides for all of your past and present help and support of me, I really appreciate it." "And Thank You all for covering my back when I needed it."

Step # 8: Then tell your Gathering, verbatim: "Please go through the bodies of all my family, and all my friends and their families, and the spiritual bodies of all my masters, guides, and ancestors and their families, and heal every part of their physical and spiritual bodies and minds."

Be sure to thank them in advance for doing this for you. This is Huge! Spiritual blessings follow willingness to help.

Step #9: Then tell your Gathering, verbatim: "Please, I need a clean and clear connection to Universal

Knowledge. This is very important to me. I want a clean and accurate connection so that when I ask things of the Universe, I get a clean and clear answer."

A very good ancient book said: "My people get not because they ask not." A word to the wise…

Promise your Gathering that you resolve to ask a lot for information that you need. Makes life much easier not having to re-invent the wheel! Be sure to thank them in advance for doing this for you.

Step # 10: Only when you are ready, do you ask your Angels to show themselves to you. You need to be ready to handle their Light and Truth, and be ready to handle your reaction to them. When you meet them ask them what future work they have for you to do. Angels often take a human form to interact with you. You blink and they are there, they deliver their message, you look away, and look back in a split second and they are gone. That's a clue.

Step # 11: Be sure to have a list of questions to ask your Angels when they come to visit. You do not want to blow the opportunity to ask them your spiritual questions. It is okay to write them down and have these questions with you and ready. You can put these questions next to your bed, and in your wallet, or simply memorize them.

Step # 12: Once you have an Angel experience, please write to this office and tell us of your encounters. We'd love to hear from you.

Step # 13: When one is ready to ask for a clearer spiritual connection with Universal Knowledge one makes this agreement with their Guides, Angels, and Ancestors: "Okay, my Gathering, listen here: I want to study the words of King David in the Psalms which he wrote as a youth. I am doing this because I want the same relationship he had with Universal Truth, and with God. When I read something in the Psalms that does not make sense to me, I want You All to make the meaning clear to me. You and I together are going on this quest. The spiritual insights should be spectacular." "I need your help on this." "Thank you all for your past help and protection."

Step # 15: Saint Ignatius of Loyola (1491-1556) Founder of the Jesuits once said; "If you don't know what to pray, simply pray; 'Thank You,' and that would be enough." A word to the wise…

Q. How can I become a super healer, and what is the purpose of all this?

A. Great Question! The purpose of doing this healing work is to rapidly handle health crisis in loved ones, and to get greater and faster healing on Earth. It will be a different world when people take greater responsibility for their health and the health of loved ones.

Never Underestimate the Power of Honoring and Respecting Your Ancestors

Step # 14: Please, Please, Please! Never underestimate the power of honoring and respecting your ancestors, Angels, Masters and guides. Their greatest fear is that they might be forgotten. Because when they are forgotten, they are forgotten for a very long time. Invite them into your daily lives, ask them for guidance, ask them to share and be a part of your daily experiences. Simply invite them along and tell them that you will never forget them, and you will tell your children and siblings to remember and honor them, too. The blessings that flow from doing this are tremendous. On a scale of one to ten, this is about an eighty-eight plus (+88+). It's really that important.

Step #15: Saint Ignatius Loyola once said: "If you don't know what to pray and you just said 'Thank You!' that would be enough." Enough said.

When Loved Ones Pass and Come to Visit

Step #16: What does one do when loved ones pass and come to visit to tell you they are fine? You talk to them just as you would in life. They are still the same. You can invite them to be with you and help you throughout your days. It is important to include them in your healing. They need healing, too. They are honored to be asked to continue to be a part of your life. And they may even help with increased blessings in your life.

Angels in the Hospital

Step #17: When you or loved ones are in the hospital it is okay to ask your Gathering to join you in your or their healing process. They appreciate being asked. There may be a DNA related connection to whatever issue you are going through and their earlier issues. It is good to clean these issues up. There are other books by this author that address spiritual and physical healing. Please get these books and read them and practice the methods taught in them.

Angels in the Corporation

There is a trend in corporations to explore the possibilities of people oriented solutions, green solutions, and spiritual solutions to business issues! This is a much needed change after five-hundred years of profits at all costs, and the "Slash and burn – scorched Earth" mentality!

When you arrive at work, why should you leave your angels and spiritual guides at the corporate door when you enter the building? Why not invite them into the building and into your cube, and occasionally into the boardroom?

Do you suppose that Angels might impact your company's bottom line?

Angels in the Cubicle

Why not put up a calendar of angel pictures in your cube?
Maybe put a few angel pictures on the opposite wall?
Maybe a few small angel statues in places around your cube? And maybe wear a small angel pin on your blouse or shirt. If these are conservatively done they should bring no objections.

If someone asks why you have angels around you could say: "I am testing to see if angels in the work place might make a difference in the company bottom line." This would make a big impact if your job was supervisory, or in company finances, or in the boardroom!

This is a small part of the info on angels, but it gives you working info on how to proceed… good experiencing! Contact us if you need any help on this.

Note: This is a companion book in the series called "Heart to Heart Healing – When you care enough to want to make a difference in the lives of loved ones." Please go to your bookstore today and buy this whole "Heart to Heart Healing series." Because the information in these books is true and it works, the information in these books is worth a thousand times what you spend on this series. This information saves you the years of research, expense, pain, and uncertainty that this author already spent getting this information for you. You and your friends need this important health-survival information. These books make the subject of healing and spirituality simple to understand. Anyone can read any of these books and immediately do the healing techniques on family and friends, and get a positive result. This makes your life much easier.

Authors Note: I talk with Angels every day and I assumed everyone knows how to do this and that they do it every day. Once I started telling people that I talk with Angels, I was amazed that they told me they don't talk with their Angels. This writing is the result of those conversations. When I am stuck as an author I ask the angels what it is I should be writing for them. I then am still and they tell me in pictures. I will get an entire chapter or book using this process. This works for me. Patience here is important. We all have gifts, and I do not deny the gifts I am given. As I discover more information I will publish it for all of you.

Frequently Asked Questions (FAQ's)

Q: "Is there anything I can do that is so bad that I would be separated from my Angels, or from Heaven?

A: One can willfully separate oneself from the realm of Angels and Heaven. This author teaches that other than willful separation, there is nothing that one can do that would separate one from Angels and Heaven. If one has been taught otherwise, so be it! There is only Love, Light, Truth, and non-judgment on the other side. Please answer this for me: "What part of Love and Truth is judgment and condemnation?" Once you have an answer to this you will be free.

Q: I don't see or feel my Angles, masters and guides. Where are they?

A: Put both of your outstretched arms behind your back. They are there at your fingertips. They are there to cover your back. You might have been looking for them in front of you.

Q: How is Shirley MacLaine? (I still get this question).
A: Shirley is fine. I talk to her every once in awhile. She continues on her spiritual journey.

Her official web site is:
http://www.shirleymaclaine.com/
She recently was awarded a Kennedy Center Honor.

Q: Is there any harm that can come from your healing processes?
A: No! There is no harm to asking your Angels for help.
And, there is no harm to bringing balance to your body's energy system.

Q. How can I become a super healer, and what is the purpose of all this?
A. Great Question! We sincerely need a shift in our health and in the health of our loved ones.
The purpose of doing this healing work is first to fix chronic pain, and to rapidly handle health crisis in loved ones, and to get greater and faster healing on Earth, and people taking greater responsibility for their health and lives.

Should Ask Questions (SAQ's):

Q: "Why would one ever want to talk with their Angels, or to ever have anything to do with them?"

A: Can you ever fathom becoming like the company that you are made in the image of, that is:
Pure Truth, Pure Light, and Pure Love? Do you suppose we can improve our connection with Our Source?
Do you suppose we can ever get our information directly from Source?
Do you suppose we can increase our collective wavelength, ever?
Do you suppose your life could possibly go better with better decision making information from an unbiased source?

If you answered "Yes" to any of the above, than this book is for you.

Prove to Me that Cell Memory is Real

About 25 years ago a little 10 year old girl needed a heart transplant. When another little girl was murdered, the girl on the transplant list got the heart of the dead girl.

The transplant girl started having these horrible nightmares of being killed. The parents sent their daughter to a psychiatrist. After months of therapy the psychiatrist concluded that this was not bad nightmares, but recall. This was because the "dream" never changed and the details were vivid. A report was sent to the police, and the person who did the murder was arrested and convicted on the heart transplant girl's information. The information in the heart was that accurate.

Sends chills down one's spine, doesn't it?
Other transplant recipients who formerly only listened to rap music, start listening to classical music. Others who had no musical talent or training would, after the transplant, take up playing the piano, flute, violin, or cello! People who had fear of heights would take up extreme rock climbing after a kidney or liver transplant. These stories are searchable on the Internet under "transplant recipient recall."

Cells do hold memory of trauma in them. This process works, and you need not believe any part of this to experience the healing from this work.

When Loved Ones Die, The Love Never Dies.
In Case You Wanted to Know

The Love never dies. When your parents, close friends, siblings, relatives die, their love never dies. Read: "Their love and care for you never dies."
Their love and care is eternal, that's what eternity is all about.
You were never abandoned when they died.
You were never told this because your teachers did not know this and they taught their "best guess." They did not tell you it was their "best guess" because they did not know. It was just the best they knew. They love you as much now as they did when they were alive. They are with you and they watch over you and they protect you. They cover your back because that is their job.
You don't believe it? Just ask them late at night and then: "Just be quiet enough to hear/see their answer." They speak in pictures. That's a clue…

Taking responsibility for the healing of your friends and family (Tribe) on a scale of one to ten is about an eighty-eight, it's that important. It dwarfs everything else one can do for their health.

There is a tsunami of false spiritual information being taught to people every day because evaluation of that information for its truth, historically, is at an all time low.

This author's job is to teach people things that work and if implemented, improves well being, health and longevity. Its all about your health and your life. As you and yours get healthier, we all get healthy around you. This is a good thing to work for.

A Bonus Book:

Book Number Two

"What did they do 100 years ago before they had all these 'Miracle Drugs?'"

Helpful Natural Tips to Stay Healthy

This is the author's opinion an is not to be considered as medical advice or treatment. Please see the disclaimer at the beginning of this book.

Rescue & Strengthen Your Compromised Immune System, a.k.a.: Hot Lemon Tea with pulp for Colds, Infection and Inflammation, etc.

Author's Opinion: Dr. Oz, Dr. Mercola, Dr. Amen, Dr. Perricone, Dr. Deepak Chopra, and others all say that inflammation is the precursor to all major diseases including cancer, stroke, and heart disease.

Read "inflammation is the precursor to all major diseases." This author has the shocking view (highly unpopular - controversial) that if a person wanted to "prevent" major diseases in their own bodies, that maybe managing inflammation in their own bodies "might" be a way to do that. Especially if one smokes and can't quit, and if one has a family history of members dying at a young age of major diseases. Now how does one do that? How can one tell if they have inflammation? Look in a mirror at your face, is it "puffy" or soft around your cheeks, or chin or throat? Touch these parts and see if they are puffy or soft. Make a fist, and look at the backs of your hands, feel them and see if they feel puffy or soft. That's inflammation, and it can be managed and controlled. By the way foods that contribute to inflammation are refined sugar, dairy, and wheat/gluten products, synthetic cooking oils, and others.

You will never see a show talking about this, except

maybe from this author. I write these things to get this healing news out to the people. "My people suffer from want of knowledge."

A note on smoking: This author believes that smoking creates a perfect environment for inflammation to take hold in the body, and creates a perfect environment for disease. Once one quits smoking your body detoxifies 50% of the smoke related poisons the first year of quitting. Each additional year your body gets rid of 50% more of the remaining toxins. There is hope…

A traditional Old World remedy for colds, infections, and inflammation, etc. given to Paul Barbaro by Dr. Ray Evers in 1995. Doctor Evers was an early founder of the Holistic Natural Foods movement in the late 1940's and early 50's. The FDA despised him and tried to stop him and his work… I wonder why? He dared to grow his own organic foods and feed them to his sick and dying patients. He paid the price for this horrible outrageous medical crime at that time with his life. This formula helps reduce infections, inflammation, and improves immune function, as well as nourishes healthy cells. This drink is not an instant healer. Rome was not built in a day. It takes time to reverse a compromised immune system. If one has a chronic health condition one needs to do this drink for at least two months every day. One gets used to the taste. Here's the recipe, it works miraculously well:

Bring to a boil 32 ounces of water in a pan on the stove. When boiling shut it off.

While it is heating up dice two medium sized lemons, skin, pulp and all and put it in the boiling water. Shut off the heat & steep for six minutes only. The hot water softens up the lemon so it blends easily. Take out the seeds because they are bitter. Do not use an aluminum pan as the acid will eat it up.

Let it cool for about ten minutes and put the entire mixture into a blender and blend until it is a smooth puree. Add honey or other sweetener because it is very bitter. You may have to add cool water to thin it down.

Drink eight ounces of this lemon tea every four hours, all day long. The cold, or infection should be gone in a few hours, or overnight at best.

Why It Works: It works because all you are doing is adding huge amounts of Vitamin C and Anti-Oxidants to your body.

The doctor told me the reason to use the pulp is because 98% of the lemon's Complex Bioflavenoids ("C – Complex") are in the pulp .

Your body's natural state is healing. When you get cut you naturally heal.

All the lemon does is boost the strength of your immune system. Lemon tea is immune support until your body can do it itself. The fact of sickness, or inflammation is proof of the compromised immune system. Vitamin C, by the way, is an antibiotic.

You can't overdose on Vitamin C or lemon juice because it's a natural food.

I have gotten so used to the taste that I no longer boil the lemon nor add sweetener.

Optional variations of this recipe: I now add two cloves of garlic, and a 2" to 4" inch ¼ inch wide strip of ginger, (Yes. Chinese style ginger.) and a 2" inch strip of fresh aloe vera (cut off the spines, and don't skin it.) and put them all in the blender with the lemon mixture. Garlic, Vitamin C and ginger are anti-bacterial, anti-inflammatory, and anti-microbial, and are antibiotic (kills invading, "bad" bacteria). This is a good thing. I hope this helps.

An Easy Gelatin Recipe to Handle Joint Pain, And Help rebuild lost cartilage.
(Jell-O = gelatin = cartilage = disks)

Every bone, joint, ligament, and cell membrane in the body contains cartilage also known as gelatin, the same as "Jell-O." Gelatin is made by boiling animal bones to get the cartilage from them. Whole Foods has a plant based, non-animal gelatin for vegans and vegetarians. Minor joint pains can be remedied by drinking a warm eight ounce gelatin mixture two times a day, for three weeks. This goes for back pain, also, as the spinal disks and knee cushioning are made of this gelatin.

When one drinks gelatin daily it strengthens joints, ligaments, muscles, cell walls, bones, nails and hair. One can not overdose on gelatin/cartilage because its food and the body will burn it as a fuel when it is not needed to strengthen body parts. A carnivore diet simply can not provide one with enough cartilage to rebuild joint cartilage.

Recipe:
Two quarts of cold water in a three quart pan,
While stirring mix in 3 – 4 heaping Tablespoons full of Knox unflavored Gelatin, get it at Smart & Final. It's about eleven dollars a pound, plus the cost of flavoring and sweetener.

While stirring mix in 3 – 4 heaping Tablespoons full of flavored Jell-O or other flavoring.

Optional: Add stevia, honey, xylitol, agave or other sweetener to taste if necessary.

Mix all the above cold, it mixes easily cold. And it does not lump.

Let it stand 5 minutes to let the crystals dissolve, then, on medium heat, heat the mixture up while stirring continuously. Do not boil, when the mixture goes "clear" in color it is ready to drink. it starts out cloudy and goes clear when luke warm.

Paul Barbaro, the healer, got this recipe in 1995 from a man that did sports injury medicine. He knew his subject. This works. Try it today, Jell-O is an inexpensive fix for mild annoying joint pain.

(Jell-O is a brand name belonging to
Illinois-based Kraft Foods)

Improved Memory and Brain Performance

In this high performance world one needs all the brain and memory power one can get. What works? Please see below.

Students and people in high-brain – memory demanding jobs need to keep sharp for a minimum of eight hours a day. B-Complex multi vitamins really help. One starts with 50 mg and later can progress to 100 mg of a good B-Complex multi vitamin. "Trader Joe's" and "Whole Foods" have decent B-Complex multi vitamins. When extremely high brain function is a must, add Niacin, 100 mgs to the B-Complex regimen. One can get a "Niacin flush" if one takes too much. This is harmless, but produces a "prickly pin" sensation all over the skin, and one can turn as red as a lobster when the blood vessels in the skin open up. Niacin is good in helping the blood carry oxygen to the brain. The brain runs on oxygen.

Caution: Caffeine triggers Niacin. Be very careful with coffee and caffeinated soft drinks until one knows how one responds to these stimulants.

By the way B-Complex and Niacin is a better way to "click the brain on" than caffeine or energy drinks. This is because caffeine and energy drinks burn up reserve vitamins and energy in the body, and one crashes due to the lack of nutrition in one's body.

Do not take Niacin nor B-Complex after 2:00 PM because it will be hard to get to sleep at night. If one can not get to sleep, melatonin and L-ornithine counteract the sleepless and "over active brain" effect.

Notes on sleep: Sleep is a powerful and critical essential "vitamin, support and nutrient" to your body and brain. One needs a minimum of five to eight hours of sleep per night. If you are really sleep deprived, it may take several days of sleep to catch up. There is no substitute for a good nights sleep.

Ginkgo Biloba and L-ornithine, an amino acid, helps memory issues. So does L-arginine.

There are two of the most powerful brain boosters on Earth. One is Oxygen, and the other is exercise. The purpose of exercise is to get Oxygen into the brain. Exercise also produces endorphins. Oxygen and exercise is so important for your brain that it dwarfs everything else. Practice inhaling through your nose and exhaling through your mouth. Exercise on a daily bases is good for circulation and good for clearing the cob webs from the brain. Exercise helps get more oxygen to the brain, as well as the rest of the body. Exercise builds muscle mass and that helps burn calories. Again the brain runs on oxygen. Your sinuses oxygenate the blood passing through your sinuses on the way to your brain. Many people are "shallow breathers." If you are a shallow breather, "Stop It. Now." You can not afford to deprive your brain of oxygen when you need all the brain power you can get.

Magnesium is a tremendous muscle relaxer. One part MgO2, magnesium oxide, and two parts calcium carbonate in warm water plus a dash of lemon makes a wonderfully relaxing drink for all times of the day. This is a blessed relief for people who can not relax. Any good "Cal-Mag" product used daily is good for relaxation. Get it at any good health or vitamin store. An inexpensive source of magnesium is Epsom salts available at any good drug store. Magnesium is involved in most of the bodies chemical reactions. It is a vital chemical. Calcium helps the magnesium to be absorbed by the cells.

Magnesium is involved in most of your body's metabolism functions. It is extremely important to get enough magnesium in your daily diet. A good inexpensive source is "Epsom Salts" which is magnesium sulfate (MgSO4). It is inexpensive and can be gotten at any drug store.

Leafy green and highly colored vegetables like carrots, beets, etc. (Raw) boost the energy producing function of your cells. These raw foods feed the macrophages within each cell that produce the energy to run the body.

Niacin & B- Complex vitamins:

L. Arginine & L. Oranthine are vital for brain function. They are essential amino acids.

L. Triptophan helps brain function. Seventy-five percent of your brain is made of L. Triptophan. A good source is cooked turkey. Supplements are available at any health or drug store.

Beliefs in Your Lifespan and Longevity

I have spoken with several people/friends who firmly believe that the length of their time here on Earth is determined by genetics, God, diet, pollution, healthy eating, etc. People tend to also believe that they can't outrun cancer or heart disease etc. even if there is a history of these diseases in their families. I am here to debunk these theories.
Your longevity can be influenced by your mind. Recent scientific studies show that thought influences and can change DNA and your genetic structure.

The Handling of Frailty

As we age we can see around us people who become frail with age. This is sad as it is so unnecessary. Can you picture your aging with as much energy as you had at age thirty-five? This is entirely possible. Your body was built for movement. When one does not move the body breaks down and frailty set in.

A One Million Dollar Cash Savings on Medical Expenses

The intent of this article is to save the reader thousands, or hundreds of thousands, or millions of dollars when one understands this data and does it.

Hospital Cost Facts: Let's say you had a major operation and the hospital sent you, or an insurance company, a bill for $250,000.00 (Two-Hundred-Fifty Thousand dollars). That's a lot of money for most people. Did you know that hospitals nationally settle these bills for four cents on the dollar with insurance companies? The hospitals over-bill so that they are paid something for their care.

Question, in disbelief: "What did you say, Paul?"
Answer: "Did you know that hospitals nationally settle these bills for four cents on the dollar with insurance companies?" They do this so that they will be paid something for the operation. Four cents on the dollar in this case would be a grand total of $10,000.00 (ten-thousand dollars). A much more affordable price for you.

Now how come every one of our politicians holler about the high cost of health care and they never mention this fact?
And, how come you spent 12 to 18 years in school and no one ever mentioned this?

Could this information save you some money in the future?
And, did you really need to sell your house, or rinance to pay the hospital?
And, can you really negotiate with your hospital and make them come to the table and give you a break on the price?
And, can you really negotiate with your hospital and make them agree to four cents on the dollar?
And doesn't that level the playing field a little in your favor?
And "Isn't that a good thing?"
And: "Do you suppose you can use this data to save money in the future?"
And: What if the hospital only lowered your bill to 25% of the original total? Would you be better off then? Can you fathom getting a break?

Fact: Most major metropolitan areas have Free Clinics that are free (!), or based on ability to pay. You may need to live in the county where these clinics are. So even if you have no money, nor insurance you can get quality care if you meet their income requirements. It is worth a phone call to find out. Google "Free Clinic" plus your zip code and see what comes up. This free care is sometimes just for serious health issues.

If you think staying healthy costs money, try illness and toxicity!

Bob Hope on Living to One Hundred Years Old

Bob Hope was once asked how he managed to live to age 100. He said that he ate a big breakfast, very little for lunch and even less for dinner. Maybe a piece of fruit or some raw vegetables. When asked "Why?" He said: "At night when I am asleep, I want my body to work on healing and purifying my system, not on digesting food!" Imagine that? Having the body heal and purify rather than digest. This seems to have worked for Bob Hope.

Author's Note: For the past two months I have tried this out. I eat a good, not heavy, breakfast, I eat a good, not heavy, lunch, and maybe an orange, an apple or a cooked yam for dinner. I am 10 pounds lighter this past month. It feels very good not carrying around that weight. I have quit all sugar, and wheat products, and that really helps. Please think about this and see if it will work for you.

Aside: George Burns was asked how he lived to 100 and he said: "I drink, I smoke, and I chase women!" Naturally he was a comedian!

An Angel Story

In the mid 1990's I used to hold "Angel Meetings" where we would invite friends over, have an informal pot luck, and share angel stories, read about angels and talk about angels. This was in Orange County in Southern California. One particular meeting I was setting up the room, and I noticed a lot of angels in the room. I asked them why they were here, because I assumed they knew all about angels. They told me "We need this information, too." So I asked them if they had friends and they said: "Yes." So I said "Bring them along, too!" The room became "packed" with angels and participants. Some of the people there noticed the angels, most did not.

After each of these meetings I would ask the people: "Are there any questions?" and the hands would go up. When I would call on people they would ask: "How do we stop hurting?" or "How do we stop the pain?"

I would get this question from one meeting to others and in frustration I asked the angels: "Why do they ask about stopping pain when I want to teach them about angels?" They said: "When they are hurting they can not focus on us (angels)." So I said: "Well 'good luck' because I know very little about getting rid of pain." The angels assured me that they would teach me how to get rid of pain. Being new at this, I wasn't too interested in this. They taught me what I needed to know and this book and this healing series are the results of this quest.

Note: These next three stories were found on the internet by this author and shared here for your enjoyment.

Breakfast at McDonald's

This is a good story and is true, please read it all the way through until the end! (After the story, there are some very interesting facts!):

I am a mother of three (ages 14, 12, 3) and have recently completed my college degree.

The last class I had to take was Sociology.

The teacher was absolutely inspiring with the qualities that I wish every human being had been graced with.

Her last project of the term was called "Smile."

The class was asked to go out and smile at three people and document their reactions.

I am a very friendly person and always smile at everyone and say hello anyway, so, I thought this would be a piece of cake, literally.

Soon after we were assigned the project, my husband, youngest son, and I went out to McDonald's one crisp March morning.
It was just our way of sharing special playtime with our son.

We were standing in line, waiting to be served, when all of a sudden everyone around us began to back away, and then even my husband did.

I did not move an inch... an overwhelming feeling of panic welled up inside of me as I turned to see why they had moved.

As I turned around I smelled a horrible "dirty body" smell, and there standing behind me were two poor homeless men.

As I looked down at the short gentleman, close to me, he was "smiling".

His beautiful sky blue eyes were full of God's Light as he searched for acceptance. He said, "Good day" as he counted the few coins he had been clutching.

The second man fumbled with his hands as he stood behind his friend. I realized the second man was mentally challenged and the blue-eyed gentleman was his salvation...

I held my tears as I stood there with them. The young lady at the counter asked him what they wanted.

He said, "Coffee is all Miss" because that was all they could afford. (If they wanted to sit in the restaurant and warm up, they had to buy something. He just wanted to be warm).

Then I really felt it - the compulsion was so great I almost reached out and embraced the little man with the blue eyes.

That is when I noticed all eyes in the restaurant were set on me, judging my every action. I smiled and asked the young lady behind the counter to give me two more breakfast meals on a separate tray. I then walked around the corner to the table that the men had chosen as a resting spot. I put the tray on the table and laid my hand on the blue-eyed gentleman's cold hand.

He looked up at me, with tears in his eyes, and said, "Thank you."

I leaned over, began to pat his hand and said, "I did not do this for you.

God is here working through me to give you hope."

I started to cry as I walked away to join my husband and son. When I sat down my husband smiled at me and said, "That is why God gave you to me, Honey, to give me hope."

We held hands for a moment and at that time, we knew that only because of the Grace that we had been given were we able to give.

We are not church goers, but we are believers.

That day showed me the pure Light of God's sweet love.

I returned to college, on the last evening of class, with this story in hand. I turned in "my project" and the instructor read it. Then she looked up at me and said, "Can I share this?" I slowly nodded as she got the attention of the class.

She began to read and that is when I knew that we as human beings and being part of God share this need to heal people and to be healed.

In my own way I had touched the people at McDonald's, my husband, son, instructor, and every soul that shared the classroom on the last night I spent as a college student.

I graduated with one of the biggest lessons I would ever learn: Unconditional acceptance. Much love and compassion is sent to each and every person who may read this and learn how to love people and to use things, not to love things and use people.

Many people will walk in and out of your life, but only true friends will leave footprints in your heart.

To handle yourself, use your head. To handle others, use your heart. God Gives every bird its food, but He does not throw it into it's nest.

A Story that Creates Hope

Throughout our lives we are blessed with spiritual experiences, some of which are very sacred and confidential, and others, although sacred, are meant to be shared. Last summer my family had a spiritual experience that had a lasting and profound impact on us, one we feel must be shared. It's a message of love. It's a message of regaining perspective, and restoring proper balance and renewing priorities. In humility, I pray that I might, in relating this story, give you a gift my little son, Brian, gave our family one summer day last year.
On July 22nd I was in-route to Washington DC for a business trip. It was all so very ordinary, until we landed in Denver for a plane change. As I collected my belongings from the overhead bin, an announcement was made for Mr. Lloyd Glenn to see the Customer Service Representative immediately. I thought nothing of it until I reached the door to leave the plane and I heard a gentleman asking every male if they were Mr. Glenn. At this point I knew something was wrong and my heart sunk. When I got off the plane a solemn-faced young man came toward me and said, "Mr. Glenn, there is an emergency at your home. I do not know what the emergency is, or who is involved, but I will take you to the phone so you can call the hospital." My heart was now pounding, but the will to be calm took over. Woodenly, I followed this stranger to the distant telephone where I called the number they gave me for the Mission Hospital. My call was put through to the trauma

center where I learned that my three-year-old son had been trapped underneath the automatic garage door for several minutes, and when my wife had found him, he was dead. CPR had been performed by a neighbor, who is a doctor, and the paramedics continued the treatment as Brian was transported to the hospital. By the time of my call, Brian was revived and they believed he would live, but they did not know how much damage was done to his brain, nor to his heart. They explained that the door had completely closed to his little sternum right over his heart. He had been severely crushed. After speaking with the medical staff, my wife sounded worried but not hysterical, and I took comfort in her calmness.

The return flight seemed to last forever, but finally I arrived at the hospital six hours after the garage door had come down. When I walked into the intensive care unit, nothing could have prepared me to see my little son laying so still on a great big bed with tubes and monitors everywhere. He was on a respirator. I glanced at my wife who stood and tried to give me a reassuring smile. It all seemed like a terrible dream. I was filled-in with the details and given a guarded prognosis. Brian was going to live, and the preliminary tests indicated that his heart was ok, two miracles in and of themselves. But only time would tell if his brain received any damage. Throughout the seemingly endless hours, my wife was calm. She felt that Brian would eventually be all right. I hung on to her words and faith like a lifeline.

All that night and the next day Brian remained unconscious. It seemed like forever since I had left for my business trip the day before. Finally at two o'clock that afternoon, our son regained consciousness and sat up uttering the most beautiful words I have ever heard spoken. He said, "Daddy hold me" and he reached for me with his little arms By the next day he was pronounced as having no neurological or physical deficits, and the story of his miraculous survival spread throughout the hospital. You cannot imagine our gratitude and joy. As we took Brian we felt a unique reverence for the life and love of our Heavenly Father that comes to those who brush death so closely. In the days that followed there was a special spirit about our home. The two older children were much closer to their little brother. My wife and I were much closer to each other, and all of us were very close as a whole family. Life took on a less stressful pace. Perspective seemed to be more focused, and balance much easier to gain and maintain. We felt deeply blessed. Our gratitude was truly profound. The story is not over (smile)!

Almost a month later to the day of the incident, Brian awoke from his afternoon nap and said, "Sit down mommy. I have something to tell you." At this time in his life, Brian usually spoke in small phrases, so to say a large sentence surprised my wife. She sat down with him on his bed and he began his sacred and remarkable story. "Do you remember when I got stuck under the garage door? Well it was so heavy and it hurt really bad. I called to you, but you wouldn't hear me. I started to cry, but then it hurt too bad. And then the birdies came." "The birdies?" my wife asked puzzled. "Yes," he replied. "The birdies made a whooshing sound and flew into the garage. They took care of me." "They did?" "Yes" he said. "One of the birdies came and got you. She came to tell you I got stuck under the door." A sweet reverent feeling filled the room. The spirit was so strong and yet lighter than air. My wife realized that a three-year-old had no concept of death and spirits, so he was referring to the beings who came to him from beyond as "birdies" because they were up in the air like birds that fly. "What did the birdies look like?" she asked. Brian answered, They were so beautiful. They were dressed in white, all white. Some of them had green and white. But some of them had on just white." "Did they say anything?" "Yes" he answered. "They told me the baby would be alright." "The baby?" my wife asked confused. Brian answered. "The baby laying on the garage floor." He went on, "You came out and opened the garage door and ran to the baby. You told the baby to stay and not leave." My wife nearly collapsed upon hearing this, for she had indeed gone and knelt beside Brian's body and seeing his crushed chest and recognizable features, knowing he was already dead, she looked up round her and whispered, "Don't leave us Brian, please stay if you can." As she listened to Brian telling her the words she had spoken, she realized that the spirit had left his body and was looking down from above on this little lifeless form. "Then what happened?" she asked. "We went on a trip." He said, "far, far away." He grew agitated trying to say the things he didn't seem to have the words for. My wife tried to calm and comfort him, and let him know it would be okay. He struggled with wanting to tell something that obviously was very important to him, but finding the words was difficult. "We flew so fast up in the air. They're so pretty Mommy." he added. "And there is lots and lots of birdies." My wife was stunned. Into her mind the sweet comforting spirit enveloped her more soundly, but with an urgency she had never before known. Brian went on to tell her that the "birdies" had told him that he had to come back and tell everyone about the "birdies". He said they brought him back to the house and that a big fire truck, and an ambulance were there. A man was bringing the baby out on a white bed and he tried to tell the man that the baby would be okay, but the man couldn't hear him. He said the birdies told him he had to go with the ambulance, but they would be near him. He said, they were so pretty and so peaceful, and he didn't want to come back. Then the bright light came. He said that the light was so bright and so warm, and he loved the bright light so much. Someone was in the bright light and put their arms around him, and told him, "I love you but you have to go back. You have to play baseball, and tell everyone about the birdies." Then the person in the bright light kissed him and waved bye-bye. Then whoosh, the big sound came and they went into the clouds. The story went on for an hour.

He taught us that "birdies" were always with us, but we don't see them because we look with our eyes and we don't hear them because we listen with our ears. But they are always there, you can only see them in here (he put his hand over his heart). They whisper the things to help us to do what is right because they love us so much. Brian continued, stating, "I have a plan, Mommy. You have a plan. Daddy has a plan. Everyone has a plan. We must all live our plan and keep our promises. The birdies help us to do that cause they love us so much." In the weeks that followed, he often came to us and told all, or part of it again and again. Always the story remained the same. The details were never changed or out of order. A few times he added further bits of information and clarified the message he had already delivered. It never ceased to amaze us how he could tell such detail and speak beyond his ability when he talked about his birdies. Everywhere he went, he told strangers about the "birdies". Surprisingly, no one ever looked at him strangely when he did this. Rather, they always got a softened look on their face and smiled. Needless to say, we have not been the same ever since that day, and I pray we never will be.

Note: This author found this story on Catholics.com in the early 2000's. It has been circulating around the Internet for years.

The Cost of a Miracle

A little girl went to her bedroom and pulled a glass jelly jar from its hiding place in the closet.

She poured the change out on the floor and counted it carefully. Three times, even. The total had to be exactly perfect. No chance here for mistakes.

Carefully placing the coins back in the jar and twisting on the cap, she slipped out the back door and made her way six blocks to Rexall's Drug Store with the big red Indian Chief sign above the door.

She waited patiently for the pharmacist to give her some attention, but he was too busy at this moment.

Tess twisted her feet to make a scuffing noise.
Nothing. She cleared her throat with the most disgusting sound she could muster. No good. Finally she took a quarter from her jar and banged it on the glass counter. That did it!

'And what do you want?' the pharmacist asked in an annoyed tone of voice... I'm talking to my brother from Chicago whom I haven't seen in ages,' he said without waiting for a reply to his question.

'Well, I want to talk to you about my brother,' Tess answered back in the same annoyed tone. 'He's really, really sick... and I want to buy a miracle.'

'I beg your pardon?' said the pharmacist.
'His name is Andrew and he has something bad growing inside his head and my Daddy says only a miracle can save him now. So how much does a miracle cost?'

'We don't sell miracles here, little girl. I'm sorry but I can't help you,' the pharmacist said, softening a little.

'Listen, I have the money to pay for it… If it isn't enough, I will get the rest. Just tell me how much it costs.'

The pharmacist's brother was a well dressed man. He stooped down and asked the little girl, 'What kind of a miracle does your brother need?'

'I don't know,' Tess replied with her eyes welling up I just know he's really sick and Mommy says he needs an operation. But my Daddy can't pay for it, so I want to use my money.'

'How much do you have?' asked the man from Chicago.
'One dollar and eleven cents,' Tess answered barely audible.

'And it's all the money I have, but I can get some more if I need to.'

'Well, what a coincidence,' smiled the man. 'A dollar and eleven cents - the exact price of a miracle for little brothers.'

He took her money in one hand and with the other hand he grasped her mitten and said 'Take me to where you live. I want to see your brother and meet your parents. Let's see if I have the miracle you need.'

That well-dressed man was Dr. Carlton Armstrong, a surgeon, specializing in neuro-surgery. The operation was completed free of charge and it wasn't long until Andrew was home again and doing well.

Mom and Dad were happily talking about the chain of events that had led them to this place.

'That surgery,' her Mom whispered. 'was a real miracle. I wonder how much it would have cost?'

Tess smiled. She knew exactly how much a miracle cost...
One dollar and eleven cents... plus the faith of a little child.

In our lives, we never know how many miracles we will need. A miracle is not the suspension of natural law, but the operation of a higher law.

How to Search Google for Health Information

Google is like a Library of Congress right at your fingertips. But a lot of people do not know how to use Google to find good free health information.

Here are some tips in Google: Type in "Natural healing diabetes." Press "Enter," and watch what comes up. You skip the first four or five search items because they want to sell you something. Then you open one article at a time and start reading. After a few articles you will see recurring themes. That is what you are going for, those recurring themes. You can copy and paste the articles that you like to a Word document and save them. I always copy and paste the URL so I can find the article again quickly. All the information is out there. You just need to know how to search for it. In Google type in:

"Natural healing memory loss."
"Natural healing diabetes."
"Natural healing stroke."
"Natural healing heart disease."
"Natural healing cancer, (breast, lung, skin, brain, etc.)"
"Natural healing fibromyalgia." Yes. Even fibromyalgia!
"Natural healing high blood pressure."
"Natural healing depression."
"Natural healing aids."
"Natural healing rosacea."
"Natural healing lupus."
"Natural healing congestive heart failure."

"Natural healing autism." Yes. Even autism.
"Natural healing epilepsy or seizures."
"Natural healing digestive-gut issues."
"Natural healing psoriasis."
"Natural healing symptoms of AIDS."
"Natural healing hair loss."
"Natural healing acne."
"Natural healing skin conditions."
"Natural healing any other conditions."

If you really want to be shocked, type in the search words at www.youtube.com.

You would be amazed to find how much information there is out there.

I am a research addict. I love research. I can't get enough of it. I love research because I can read a study that gives me fabulous information and I did not have to spend money on for that research! What a windfall! There are great published research works that nobody knows about and they are out there for me to find. Valuable healing studies and information. The healthier your community is, the healthier you tend to be.

A Good Book once said: "My people suffer for want of knowledge."

And: *"My people get not because they ask not."* And St. James 4:2 Says: *"We have not because* we *ask not."*

Notes on Cancer and Major Diseases
Fixing Your Compromised Immune System

Note: There is no suggestion here that this is medical advice nor that anyone should do any of this without their medical doctor's permission.

Cancer is a tragic diagnosis. I have lost several close best friends, family members, and relatives to cancer. My cancer research started in 1995 when I lost a beloved younger sister, Mary, 15 years younger than I, to cancer.
Cancer, AIDS, and other life threatening diseases are evidence of a compromised immune system.
Sugar feeds cancer, so does sodas with artificial sweeteners. So as a start avoid all sugars and artificial sweeteners in all their forms. Because wheat products convert to sugar when digested, restrict as much as possible gluten and wheat products. When one stops feeding the cancer cells they tend to die off and half the battle is won. Some sweeteners like Xylitol have anti-bacterial properties. Use Xylitol.

Cancer cells can not live in the body when the blood pH is above 7.2 . At a blood pH of 7.2 your immune system clicks "On" and your body kills the cancer cells and other invading bacteria and viruses. It is worth having a strong immune system to fight disease before it ever takes hold. To raise blood pH one can add ½ teaspoon of soda bicarbonate to a glass of water and drink it 2 to 3 times a day. If you can taste the soda bicarbonate you are using too much. Eating lemon and watermelon, and using apple cider vinegar daily also raises blood pH! They go in as an acid and they turn base when it hits the stomach. Get online and research this. Urine and saliva pH has nothing to do with Blood pH. Have your doctor check your blood pH with every blood test.

Note: When one has a blood panel of tests ask your doctor to check blood pH, also. There is no relationship between blood pH, urine pH, and saliva pH. One can check urine pH, and saliva pH, but it has nothing to do with blood pH.

Vitamin D-3 by all medical studies is very tough on cancer cells.
Raw Garlic is hell on cancer cells. So is raw ginger.
So is doing coffee enemas (brewed strong and then cooled down, of course!)
They detoxify the colon, and get poisons out of the body.

One can "Google" "Natural cure for cancer" and read all the articles that come up. After reading ten articles, a common theme will emerge. That's what you are looking for.

When one's doctor finally says: "Go home and get your affairs in order, you have six weeks to live." Only then do people call and go to the Gerson Institute in San Diego, California. (www.gerson.com) The Gerson

Institute has been naturally curing cancer for over thirty years. My clients tell me that they would: "Rather die than change my diet to eat naturally, or do their other suggestions!"

Author's note: I am not so stubborn that I would prefer death to changing my diet, or to do their other suggestions. Also, when the Gerson Institute can reverse cancer within six weeks of death, why not go a year or two before it's terminal??? What a strange concept? Why would one ever want to live a long, pain, disease free and happy-healthy life?

Either you are going to take your health in your own hands, or you are going to give up and die. I'd rather live, I have a lot of valuable work to do and there are still a lot of things I would like to do before I die. End of authors note.

There is a Native American Shaman named Robert Roy a.k.a. "Two Feathers" that has an ancient Native American healing formula that works very well on cancer. I know him
personally, and I trust his products.
http://www.healingformula.net/
robert@healingformula.net   His Phone: (775) 324 - 4889

Caroline Sutherland, a "Medical Intuitive," has cancer information resources. It is worth reading. This following section is copied and pasted from Caroline's web site: http://carolinesutherland.com/resources.cfm

Useful resources:

Do not consume the following items all at once.

Pau d'Arco tea – a medicinal tea from South America. Three to six cups a day may be useful.

Essiac tea – a combination herb formula originally from Canada thought to be useful for cancer – one to four ounces per day.

Elixer Vitale - A doctor whose opinion I respect suggested this potent herbal formula. I have had no experience with this item.

Call Caroline Sutherland for more information
307 266-5310.

There are many clinics with unusual treatments for cancer. Tijuana, Mexico abounds with such places. You also might want to research Klinik St. Georg in Bad Aibling, Germany. Check their website at www.klinik-st-georg.de
or other treatments at:
www.alternativemedicine.com   subheading "cancer"

Contemporary Medicine and Insulin Potentiation Therapy: A Renaissance in Cancer Chemotherapy. Insulin Potentiation Therapy (IPT)
(www.iptforcancer.com) is a new approach to the

challenge of cancer that involves no new drug products, but simply the innovative use of some old ones. Taking advantage of the very mechanisms that cancer has developed to promote its own growth, IPT employs the hormone insulin to selectively target lowered doses of anticancer drugs into the cancer cells, with a reduced or complete absence of drug side effects. Thus these powerful cell-killing chemotherapy drugs may now be used in a much safer manner. Combined with this kinder and gentler medical treatment, we provide help with education and inspiration in the areas of Nutrition and Mind-Body Medicine.

Please note: I, Caroline Sutherland accept no responsibility for the health of any individual following the above suggestions. Seek the advice of your medical doctor before implementing any program.
- End of Caroline Sutherland's article.

More Cancer Notes

Cancer Update: I have heard there is an alternative to chemotherapy.

1. Every person has cancer cells in their body. These cancer cells do not show up in the standard tests until they have multiplied to a few billion. When doctors tell cancer patients that there are no more cancer cells in their bodies after treatment, it just means the tests are unable to detect the cancer cells because they have not reached the detectable size/number.

2. Cancer cells occur between six to more than ten times in a person's lifetime.

3. When the person's immune system is strong the cancer cells will be destroyed and prevented from multiplying and forming tumors. A compromised immune system is an easy target for cancer cells.

4. When a person has cancer it indicates the person has multiple nutritional deficiencies. These could be due to genetic, environmental, food and/or lifestyle factors.

5. To overcome the multiple nutritional deficiencies, changing diet and including supplements will strengthen the immune system.

6. Chemotherapy involves poisoning the rapidly-growing cancer cells and also destroys rapidly-growing healthy cells in the bone marrow, gastro-intestinal tract etc, and can cause organ damage, like liver, kidneys, heart, lungs etc. In other words, chemotherapy compromises an already compromised immune system.

7. Radiation while destroying cancer cells also burns, scars and damages healthy cells, tissues and organs.

8. Initial treatment with chemotherapy and radiation will often reduce tumor size. However prolonged use of chemotherapy and radiation do not result in more tumor destruction.

9. When the body has too much toxic burden from chemotherapy and radiation the immune system is either compromised or destroyed, hence the person can succumb to various kinds of infections and complications. The treatment has risks/dangers.

10. Chemotherapy and radiation can cause cancer cells to mutate and become resistant and difficult to destroy. Surgery can also cause cancer cells to spread to other sites.. I have asked many doctors how one cures cancer by compromising the immune which is the body's natural defense system? Their answer was that the immune system is already compromised by the cancer. My view is why not build a strong immune system so one can fight cancer naturally. I believe we can change our habits for

the benefit of better health when that is a priority in our lives.

11. An effective way to battle cancer is to starve the cancer cells by not feeding it with the foods it needs to multiply.

Cancer cells feed on:

12. Sugar, it feeds cancer.
By cutting off sugar it cuts off one important food supply to the cancer cells. Sugar substitutes like Nutra-Sweet, Equal, Spoonful, etc are made with Aspartame and it is harmful. A better natural substitute would be Manuka honey or molasses but only in very small amounts. Table salt has a chemical added to make it white in color. Better alternative is Bragg's amino or sea salt.

13. Milk causes the body to produce mucus, especially in the gastro-intestinal tract. Cancer feeds on mucus. By cutting off milk and substituting with unsweetened soya milk cancer cells are being starved.

14. Cancer cells thrive in an acid environment.
A meat-based diet is acidic and it is best to eat fish, and a little organic chicken rather than beef or pork. Meat also contains livestock antibiotics, growth hormones and parasites, which are all harmful, especially to people with cancer.

15. A diet made of 80% fresh vegetables and juice, whole grains, seeds, nuts and a little fruit helps put the body into an alkaline environment. About 20% can be from cooked food including beans. Fresh vegetable juices provide live enzymes that are easily absorbed and reach down to cellular levels within 15 minutes to nourish and enhance growth of healthy cells. To obtain live enzymes for building healthy cells try and drink fresh vegetable juice (most vegetables including bean sprouts) and eat some raw vegetables 2 or 3 times a day. Enzymes are destroyed at temperatures of 104 degrees F (40 degrees C) and above.

16. Avoid coffee, tea, and chocolate, which have high caffeine. Green tea is a better alternative and has cancer-fighting properties. Water- it is best to drink purified water, or filtered, to avoid known toxins and heavy metals in tap water.

17. Meat protein is difficult to digest and requires a lot of digestive enzymes. Undigested meat remaining in the intestines become putrefied and leads to more toxic build-up. Toxicity and poisons reduce the effectiveness of the immune system. Your immune system is a digestive system. It attacks, kills and digests invading bacteria. Then the poisons are cleaned from the body by the liver and kidneys.

18. Cancer cell walls have a tough protein covering. By refraining from or eating less meat it frees more enzymes

to attack the protein walls of cancer cells and allows the body's killer cells to destroy the cancer cells.

19. Some supplements build up the immune system (IP6, Floressence, Essiac, anti-oxidants, vitamins, minerals, EFAs etc.) to enable the body's own killer cells to destroy cancer cells. Other supplements like vitamin E are known to cause apoptosis, or programmed cell death, the body's normal method of disposing of damaged, unwanted, or unneeded cells.

20. Cancer is a disease of the mind, body, and spirit. A proactive and positive spirit will help the cancer warrior be a survivor. This author is a big proponent of forgiveness. Anger, un-forgiveness and bitterness put the body into a stressful and acidic environment. Learn to have a loving and forgiving spirit. Learn to relax and enjoy life.

21. Cancer cells cannot thrive in an oxygenated environment. Exercising daily, and deep breathing help to get more oxygen down to the cellular level. Oxygen therapy is another means employed to destroy cancer cells. Some people go to Mexico for intravenous peroxide therapy for killing cancer cells. More than one person has walked five miles a day to get exercise and to put oxygen into their bodies. They are still cancer free 15 years later.

22. There has been more than one person who laughed their way out of cancer. They rented dozens of comedy movies and spent a month watching them and laughing hard. One month later they had no cancer. Laughter produces endorphins.

Additional Health Tips:

No plastic containers nor plastic wrap in microwave. They produce PCB's. (Polychlorinated Biphenyls). www.epa.gov/osw/hazard/tsd/pcbs/about.htm

No water bottles in freezer. They produce dioxin and oxytocin.

Dioxin chemicals causes cancer, especially breast cancer. Dioxins are highly poisonous to the cells of our bodies. Don't freeze your plastic bottles with water in them as this releases dioxins from the plastic.

Recently, Dr. Edward Fujimoto, Wellness Program Manager at Castle Hospital was on a TV program to explain this health hazard. He talked about dioxins and how bad they are for us. He said that we should not be heating our food in the microwave using plastic containers. This especially applies to foods that contain fat. He said that the combination of fat, high heat, and plastics releases dioxin into the food and ultimately into the cells of the body.

Instead, he recommends using glass, such as Corning Ware, Pyrex or ceramic containers for heating food. You get the same results, only without the dioxin.

So such things as TV dinners, instant ramen and soups, etc., should be removed from the container and heated in something else. Paper isn't bad but you don't know what is in the paper. It's just safer to use tempered glass, Corning Ware, ceramic, etc. He reminded us that a while ago some of the fast food restaurants moved away from the foam containers to paper. The dioxin problem is one of the reasons. Also, he pointed out that plastic wrap, such as Saran, is just as dangerous when placed over foods to be cooked in the microwave. As the food is nuked, the high heat causes poisonous toxins to actually melt out of the plastic wrap and drip into the food. Cover food with a paper towel instead.

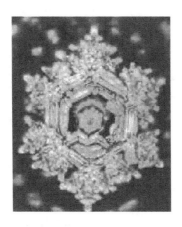

Dr. Masaru Emoto's Messages From Water

Author's Note: Your body is 80% water. And every molecule of water on earth follows the cycles of the sun and moon. That's why this study is relevant.

As someone who devotes his life to helping others learn to use prayer and blessing to improve their lives, I am intrigued and inspired by Dr. Masaru Emoto's work. As a dowser, I am naturally fascinated with water. Dr. Emoto had long wondered if there were methods of expressing difference in the nature of water. He knew that water from a natural spring, for example, was better for you than tap water or stagnant water. When Dr. Emoto read in a children's book that no two snowflakes have the same shape, he thought that the same thing must apply to frozen water crystals. Dr. Emoto wondered if he could develop a way to photograph frozen water crystals. Does water have messages for us? Can we develop ways to receive those messages from water?

So after much trial and error, Dr. Emoto developed a process in which he would freeze drops of water and take photographs of individual water crystals that formed. He found that his theory was correct: like snowflakes, every water crystal is unique. But he learned much more than that. Dr. Emoto found that you could tell much about the nature of the water by photographing it in this way, and more importantly, that, as human beings, we can change the nature of water in many ways. Water truly does have powerful messages for us.

One of the first things that Dr. Emoto learned was that all water does not form beautiful crystals. He tested tap water from around the world and found that tap water does not form water crystals. Stagnant or polluted water does not form water crystals either, but forms unpleasant, deformed frozen structures. Rainwater, water from clean streams and rivers, water from glaciers, and water from holy places around the world form beautiful crystals when frozen.

Then he wondered if we, as human beings, can change the nature of water, so he tried many techniques to test this. Dr. Emoto found that if he played beautiful music in the presence of tap water, it would then make beautiful frozen crystal formations. He also learned that the written word changed the water. Dr. Emoto taped paper strips on bottles of tap water and then photographed the frozen water. He found that words such as "Thank you," and "I love you," caused the tap water to form beautiful crystals (see picture at left). Words such as "You make me sick," or "You are a fool," caused ugly, distorted crystals or no crystals at all. Dr. Emoto then found that we can cause tap water to form beautiful frozen water crystals simply by praying for the water, by sending it loving thoughts, and by blessing it.

Bonus: On the next page are labels that you can copy and tape to your water jug, glass, bottle, and or container.
You can step and repeat them and make several at a time.

LOVE	LOVE
JOY	JOY
PEACE	PEACE
GRATITUDE	GRATITUDE
SERENITY	SERENITY
CONNECTION	CONNECTION
BLESSINGS	BLESSINGS
MEDITATION	MEDITATION
FORGIVENESS	FORGIVENESS
PROSPERITY	PROSPERITY
HEALING	HEALING
ABUNDANCE	ABUNDANCE
THANK YOU!	THANK YOU!

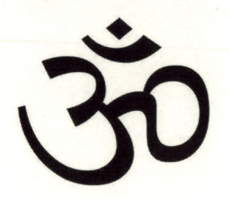 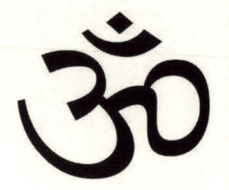

How Can I Tell If I Am Dehydrated?

Dehydration is epidemic in our society. Dehydration impairs healthy functions. Your body is 80% water, and water is essential to keep toxins flushing out of your body.
Dehydration is a low level of water in the body. Lower than normal for optimum bodily functioning. Ones body can take a lot of abuse before symptoms show up. This is problematic as we are not taught to connect dots.
How can I tell if I am dehydrated?
Do you drink a lot of coffee or alcohol, and not a lot of water?
Then you are probably dehydrated.
Do you wake up at night and your mouth or eyes are as dry as cotton? You are probably dehydrated.
Is your pee dark orange or brown in the morning? You are probably dehydrated.

The Remedy

When you find that you are dehydrated, drink about half a gallon of water more per day than you drink now.
Re-hydration is not an instant process. It takes awhile, be patient and drink a lot of water. Have you ever heard: "My People Suffer for Want of Knowledge…" A word to the wise… This information works.
Drinking coffee and alcohol is OK as long as you know it is dehydrating you, and you take appropriate re-hydrating

action. Willfully staying dehydrated is asking for disaster. This author's research leads him to believe that dehydration is a contributing factor in stroke and heart disease. A word to the wise… Stay hydrated.

It takes about three days or more of drinking a lot of water to totally re-hydrate one's body. Then don't quit drinking that amount of water each day.
Acidic water helps acidify your body. Increased body acidity promotes disease and death.
Every (All) of those store bought waters like "Crystal Geyser" are 3.0 pH. Do not drink them because they are hugely acidic and they acidify your body. Get your litmus strips and test them. Also, test all soda type soft drinks. It is shocking how acidic those store bought waters and soft drinks are.

The Dangers of A Low Blood pH

An acidic blood pH promotes diseases like cancer. A blood pH lower than 7.2 can cause a rapidly growing cancer to kill you in sixty days. Do you ever wonder how those friends or relatives, or siblings had a clean bill of health, and a few months later they were dead? I truly wonder why you were never told this information. Correct knowledge and prevention is a blessing. Next time your doctor does a blood panel, ask them to do blood pH also. The test is inexpensive and gives you an idea where you are pH wise. Eating raw green vegetables tend to raise blood pH.

How the Buddha Achieved Enlightenment

Imagine with me for a minute what the U.S.A. would be like if each state in the union had five enlightened beings like the Buddha walking around helping people, meditating, glowing with enlightenment, teaching and radiating peace, connection, and centered-ness to all. I'm suggesting that the emotional and spiritual energy of each state might be much different. Do you suppose that our destructive weather patterns might change for the better? Do you suppose that it would be harder for terrorist groups to attack America and Americans? Maybe we might not need to print money to buy dictators and wars? Maybe we wouldn't need to deliberately cause wars to get our oil, or to have a nice comfortable retirement plan(!) ?
I'm not trying to make a political statement here, but to invite you to please join me in pondering these wonderful possibilities!

Mother Theresa & Ghandi

Mother Theresa, and Ghsandi once said; "You must be the change you want to see in the world." Is it possible to produce an American who cares enough about their future to decide to put down their TV's, entertainment centers, video games, cell/i-phones, I-pads, mobile devices, and unplug from the digital world long enough to be the change they want to see in the world? And to commit to do this process?

Do you suppose that we could get a few of our unemployed college graduates to decide and commit to do the "Buddha making process" and become enlightened just on the chance that their lives, their families, and their communities might suddenly change for the better? Or what if a few bored retired seniors decided that now they can take the time to do something more productive with their time/lives and do the "Buddha making process?" Why not take the abundance of our human resources into consideration?

The Precise, Exact, Step-by-Step Buddha Making Process:

When one sees a statue of the Buddha one sees the exact process he went through to become enlightened. One has to read into it to get the message.

He knew exactly what he was doing when he sat under the Bodhi tree so long ago. The statue is your lesson for how to attain enlightenment for yourself. Enlightenment comes from within, and it is a connection to and with Universal mind.

The first thing the Buddha did was to have a burning desire to become enlightened. He was aware that such a state existed. He had tried being an acetic for years. For years he would eat a single grain of rice per meal as his only food. He did drink lots of water. He would punish his body to discipline himself. He found that this was not working. After a lifetime of trying everything else that did not work, this is what the Buddha did;

Buddha sat on the ground his back was against the Bodhi tree. He grounded himself and his eyes were closed for forty days and forty nights. He was determined to do the process for as long as it takes.

(What if it had taken him 50 days? Or how about 60 days? Would that have been worth it?)

Once grounded he became an antenna for receiving Universal truth. He assumed the lotus position. He knew that the pineal gland is the connection between the body and Universal Mind. He knew that the pineal gland, in the center of the head, is activated by darkness. Buddha might have worn a head band or a blindfold to keep the light out. He had a group of dedicated friends bring him food and water, He did not care if it rained or shined! The rain would make a better grounding connection for him to be a human antenna for the wisdom of the Universe. The Bodhi tree is key here, also. The tree is an antenna and it's roots are in the ground (grounded). The tree also shaded direct light from the Buddha's eyes and protected him from the sun. Do you remember in the movie "Avitar?" The trees were connected to the planet and to each other and they supported healing and grounding.

Buddha meditated and kept his eyes closed for forty days and forty nights. Some texts have different number of days.
In Western religious writings, forty days and forty nights is repeated several times as being spiritually significant. In the story of Noah and the Arc it rained for forty days and forty nights. People would fast in the desert for forty days and forty nights in order to kill parasites in their bodies. The boy David killed Goliath after the giant insulted the God of Israel for forty days and forty nights.
The apostles were in the upstairs windowless room (it was dark*) for forty days and forty nights, then the Pentecost took place. Pentecost could be likened to enlightenment. The apostles knew what they were doing, as did Christ. And there are other stories of similar time periods. Do you remember that the Buddha continued to meditate after he was enlightened?

Note: * The pineal gland in the center of your brain is activated by darkness.

Grounding is one-third of the process. Meditating is one-third of the process. And commitment is the other one-third. Commitment is the intense desire to do all the work required to achieve results.

Centers of Light

The way these enlightenment centers, or "Centers of Light" would work would be an extensive interview process to select candidates, based on service to family and community or to the nation. The center would have rooms for all life's basic functions. Such as bed rooms for sleeping, with grounded beds so during sleep a candidate can maintain their grounding. There would be dark dining rooms and dark bathrooms. There could be attendants that would guide the candidates around. There could be tiny dim green or red lights around (like in a dark room) that put a minimum amount of non-interfering light in the rooms. There could be many trees planted in the meditation rooms for leaning against while meditating, with well grounded floors. The trees would grow through the roof, and all light below the ceiling would be blocked out. All candidates needs would be met. Movement would be kept to a minimum. Part of their meditation would be focus on breathing. Each candidate would sign a pledge to not sneak a peek at light, or "chip" on light for at least "X" number of days.

Such a center would need a continuous stream of money to continue operations. After a good reputation is established for this center, candidates would apply from all over the world. Do you suppose that would produce a global shift? Do you suppose it would be worth your time helping raise money for such a center? Do you know anyone who would like to join us in this effort? Please let us know. (408) 253-6577 Ask for Paul Barbaro, director.

Healing Principals:

1). There is a spiritual side to a person and to their body, we are spiritually connected to each other by universal energy,
2). The body heals faster when the spirit and one's angels, ancestors, guides and family are considered during the healing process. We call this one's "Tribe."
3). The spirit of each person is energetically connected to their ancestors, guides, angels, families, friends and masters,
4). That when this spiritual community is included in healing, the recovery is quicker, more stable, and longer lasting,
5). That a major part of holistic (whole) healing is including ones "Tribe" into the healing process.
6). 100% of all modern medicine is based on the patient being just a chunk of meat that has a medical condition. And for every symptom there is an appropriate drug or surgery to fix that issue. This needs to change.
7). The spirit of each person shares the same rights as that person. They are inseparable.
8). Can we ever fathom that there is a spirit?
9). Can we ever fathom the spirit having rights?
10). Can we ever fathom the spirit being recognized and honored in this country U.S.A.?

11). Can we ever fathom the spirit can improve?
12). Can we ever fathom the spirit being an integral part of our healing process?
14). Can we ever fathom the spirit being an integral part of our daily lives?
15). Add your own hopes and prayers here, _____.

There is a life force in the body, and that force can be strong or weak. And just like muscle, life force can be increased. It can become so strong that it is unstoppable. Early childhood pain can compromise one's immune system.

Throughout my journey I have come back to realize that true knowledge can only be uncovered from within myself; balanced by mind, body and spirit, driven by my hearts conscious expression for love towards all things.

Ultimately, my true purpose is to move into and with the true frequencies of our natural cosmic universe, using heart as my compass and engine. Still I continue to research, practice and transpose with such passion. Love is my work and my passion. Love is so close to Light that they seem to be the same. There is only one Light and one Truth (capital "T"). All Truth aligns with all other Truth. This makes your life much easier when seeking Truth. If it does not align with other Truths, it probably is not true.

How to Re-Colonize Your Gut with Good Bacteria

This author is only interested in things that work. This works extremely well. Try it and see if it works for you. You just need to do it. You must check with a competent medical professional before doing any of these suggestions.

Preface: We people, as a species tend to be constipated most the time. I get four calls a month from friends and others that have constipation. Fiber is the remedy to handling constipation. But how does one get fiber in a pleasant form? There are two products that are easy to use and add fiber to your gut. They are "Miralax," and "Fiber Gummies" by "VitaFusion." Yes! "Fiber Gummies!" They work. Both are at Costco and most drug stores. A community of support for one's health is good to build.

Even though antibiotics are needed when the immune system is compromised, they do kill off the good bacteria in the gut. Excessive gas and bloating, poor digestion, and cramps and pains after a meal tend to be indications of a lack of good bacteria in the gut. One can eat bowls of yogurt, but the stomach acid kills most the good bacteria.

So what to do? One can take those small little pills that bypass the stomach and dissolve in the small intestine. Takes two weeks to a month of taking these pills.

An enema of probiotics (yogurt) can help. One first does a small water enema just to clean out the colon and rectum. Then mix a heaping tablespoon full of a good plain yogurt, no fruit or flavoring, in a half-cup of warm water. "Trader Joe's," "Whole Foods" and most grocery stores have good plain yogurt. Mix it well and if it is too thick, thin it with more water. Make sure all of your equipment is sterile! Sterilize with alcohol, ammonia, hydrogen peroxide, or with great care, a 10% mixture of water and Clorox. Put only two to four ounces of this mixture into you at a time. There will be a feeling of pressure and a desire to expel it immediately. Resist the feeling and try to hold it in for at least an hour. If you expel the mixture before 10 minutes, you should do it again, and try to hold that for an hour. Do this every other day for two weeks. Never mix chlorine and ammonia as it produces a deadly gas.

Key: Your colon and your small intestines know what to do with these friendly bacteria probiotics. When the good bacteria get absorbed they "Colonize" in the gut. They reproduce and thrive until they get killed off again. This is the key. One should feel more energy and better digestion in two days after doing this. Your stools may change color. You may go through a detox reaction, that is, putrefied waste coming out of you for a day or two. To be sure of full colonization, do this every other day for two weeks. If you are currently on antibiotics you may need to do this daily.

Key: Your immune system is a digestive system. You have a strong immune system when you have a strong digestive system. My sources for this information are Dr. George Carr, M.D., and Dr. Ray Evers, M.D.. The reason you have not heard of this is because the establishment can not make tons of money doing this. This works very well.

Please contact this office if you see no improvements after two weeks.

Testimonial: "Using Paul's materials, this is the first time in years that I feel really clean, inside and out."
– Mark W.

This is provided as educational, informational, and entertainment purposes only. Always seek the advice of a competent medical professional before doing any of this.

Handling Your Enemies with Feng Shui

Whenever I write about ways to warm the hearts of enemies and those who might wish you harm, I get tremendous response. Today, here's another technique to take the sting out of an angry relationship. To sweeten someone's disposition towards you just write their name in green in a slip of white paper. Now put that paper into any small glass jar that has a lid. Completely cover the paper with honey and seal the jar tightly shut. Place a small white tea candle atop the jar to burn, visualizing the enmity between the two of you going up in smoke. Put this jar anywhere inside the 'Family/Friends/Ancestors' area, and leave it there for 27 days. After that, you can dispose of the jar any way you see fit, and your friction should be long gone.

Educators around the globe are celebrated today on World Teacher Day. As a mom to a young schoolboy myself, I am often asked by his savvier teachers if there is anything from the world of Feng Shui that might enhance the learning energy in the classroom, and that answer is a resounding 'Yes!' First, and most importantly, it is critical to clear the clutter in the classroom -- always easier said than done. But even just tackling one small file cabinet and getting that in order will improve the classroom energy as a whole. Rearrange desks so that they are not in a straight line. Embracing a curvilinear architectural bent inside this room will also encourage creativity and thinking outside the box. Also try to keep some healthy green plants. Not only will these bring fresh oxygen and Chi to the classroom, but will also foster a sense of health and healing as well. We honor and love our teachers, and we offer gratitude for all that they do.

This Author's Guarantee to You:

Besides continuing to give you workable healing methods, and my commitment to relentless research for healthy things that work, I guarantee that I will give you technical support on this healing system as long as you need it. Call me before you do a group meeting and tell me you need support on a certain day and between certain times. When you call I will be there for you to answer any questions. There is no need to stay stuck! (408) 253-6577, Our healing center is in Cupertino, California, U.S.A., near Apple Computer.

What this Author Needs from You!

Most communities have movers and shakers that are working to make people better. Please find the five most active community leaders in your area and give them a copy of this book. Please ask them to do the process with their groups. Please, also take this process into your communities and where ever you can gather a group of people, churches, community organizations, clubs, family and friends gatherings, reunions, etc.. Please use this process to heal them. As your communities heal, the collective energy of this world will shift. When we reach the critical mass, like the "Hundredth Monkey," then our society's consciousness will shift and real global healing will take place. Maybe we can build a better world for ourselves and for our children.

The intention behind this book is to get copies into the hands of the national representatives at the United Nations in New York. This intention can also be extended to all leaders as well as all governing bodies. This author believes that when these leaders take this healing method to their own countries, and they do the process regularly, we collectively can produce the needed healing shift much faster. People wishing to contribute to this campaign are welcome to contact this office and we can discuss the possibilities. We also need volunteers.

Please also buy ten copies of this book and give them to community and church leaders, as well as healers and people in the wellness professions. This will help in the push to get this information out into the world.

If you are good at proofreading or editing, and you send me a marked up copy of this book, as long as the suggestions are significant, I will mail you five (5) books in return. I can really use your help on this. This offer is good now and for up to one year from March 1, 2014.

This author is "Social Media Challenged."

This author is "Social Media Challenged." Please post news of this healing process on Twitter, Facebook, Tumblr, Instagram Pinterest, Linkedin, Pinterest, Google Plus, and even MySpace, Tagged, and all the others, and create buzz and awareness.

If you wish to donate your time to help this organization we can use all the help we can get. This is a volunteer position because we have a limited budget. Donating money, cars, and/or real estate is also appreciated and the funds keep us working.

Working on a PBS Special

You are a gold mine of ideas! I need ideas for this PBS special to present this process to the world!
If you have any ideas for this PBS special, please jot them down for me and email them to this office. Please be sure to add your name, email address and phone number. Our **email address** is: **healingangelguides@yahoo.com:**

Also, we are targeting a budget for this special of $250,000. We need all the donations we can get to create this special. We have a creative team in place ready to produce this special. We just need the funds.

I Need Ideas for These:

- A title for this PBS Special about community healing
- A book title to accompany this PBS Special
- A title for a book about Angels
- A title for a book about honoring and healing Ancestors

Thank You for your help on this.

Permission to Copy this Book

There is bulk pricing available from this office that is lower than the cost of copying. Our intention is to get this work out into the world and to be widely used. Please call this office for bulk pricing.

Permission to copy this book is based on several conditions being met. Please call this office for further information, **(408) 253-6577** and tell us of your intention to do that.

Otherwise: All rights reserved.

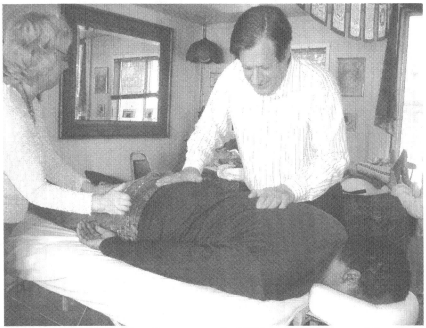

This photo is of our healing center in Willow Glen, part of San Jose, California. In the photo is Paul Barbaro, his wonderful assistant Mona Angel, and a client named Robert.

Bio of author, Paul Barbaro

Paul Barbaro is an author of four books, speaker, health researcher, and longevity coach. He studied Psychology, languages, education and has a BS degree from UC Riverside, California.

Paul is an "Angel Whisperer." Paul channels your angels to help in your healing. He is an avid medical researcher. His strength is that he knows what he is looking for and does not quit until he finds it. Paul's persistence keeps him looking only for those things that work consistently well. Paul's healing system was given to him by two Native American (First Nation) Indian shamans. Paul had a thriving healing practice in 2008, and when he added this healing system to his practice, his healing results and client satisfaction went through the roof!

Mr. Barbaro has said: "Throughout my journey I have come back to realize that true knowledge can only be uncovered from within myself; balanced by mind, body and spirit, driven by my hearts conscious expression for love towards all things.

Ultimately, my true purpose is to move into and with the true frequencies of our natural cosmic universe, using heart as my compass and engine. Still I continue to research, practice and transpose with such passion. Love is my work and my passion. Love is so close to Light that they seem to be the same. There is only one Light and one Truth (capital "T"). All Truth aligns with all other Truth. This makes your life much easier when seeking Truth. If it does not align with other Truths, it probably is not true."

Paul continues his research and healing work in Cupertino, California, near Apple Computer, and people interested in Paul's healing magic can call and make appointments. One does need to come to California, and stay for awhile. Healers that have a practice or spa can learn to do this healing system and boost their results and client satisfaction. There are training classes available in California. Paul presents informative, entertaining, enlightening, and captivating talks, lectures and presentations! Please call to book Mr. Barbaro for your next event.

Our Donation Hotline Phone Number:

1 (408) 253-6577

We can accept donations from all over the United States. We can use cars, SUV's, trucks, real estate, trusts, stock and trading accounts, boats, RV's, timeshares, jewelry, coin and stamp collections, antiques, and anything of value. We are applying for tax exempt status and we appreciate your support and donations. Please use this number for donations only as each call costs us money.

Thank you for buying and reading this book. It is important to get this information out into the teal world.

It is okay with us for you to buy ten copies or more of this book and give them out to friends, family members, people in the healing arts and total strangers. For deep discounts on large orders, please call this office because we can sell the books lower than the list price. I hope this helps.

Thank You.

Sincerely,

Paul Barbaro, Health Author

Made in the USA
Charleston, SC
30 July 2016